Elizabeth and her Extra X

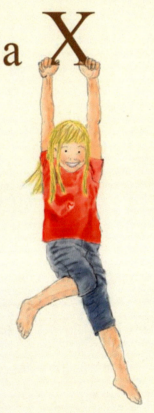

Copyright 2014 Regents of the University of Colorado.
All Rights Reserved

Created by Arlene Colvin, Suzanne Hayes, Susan Howell, and Nicole Tartaglia.

All characters appearing in this work are fictitious. Any resemblance to real persons, living or dead, is purely coincidental.

Forward

The inspiration for the creation of this book comes from working with the families of children with X&Y chromosome variations both in the eXtraordinarY Kids Clinic and at family conferences around the world. There were so many times that we handed reading materials and textbook chapters to parents to learn more about their child's condition, while we had nothing to give their smart, curious children standing next to them. Also, parents often ask how to discuss the diagnosis with their child, but feel unprepared and ill-equipped to do so. This book was created to allow girls with Triple X to learn more about their condition, and to facilitate the discussion between parents and their child about the diagnosis of Triple X.

The author, Arlie Colvin, and the illustrator, Suzanne Hayes, have taken a complex topic and created a fantastic story that explains features of Triple X in a way that kids will be able to understand. Elizabeths's day captures the story of so many girls we see in the clinic--both children and parents will relate to her experiences. Truly understanding the diagnosis of Triple X takes more than a diagram of chromosomes and can't be fully described by a medical textbook, and this book now provides that missing piece. We look forward to using this book as a tool to support girls with Triple X and their families both today and in the years to come.

Nicole Tartaglia, MD

Susan Howell, MS, CGC

eXtraodinarY Kids Clinic
Children's Hospital Colorado
University of Colorado School of Medicine

Recommendations for using this resource.

Many parents of children with X&Y chromosome variations (also called sex chromosome aneuploidy or sex chromosome abnormalties) report feeling unprepared to talk with their child about the diagnosis. Most parents and adult individuals with X&Y chromosome variations say the discussion should happen early in life. It is our hope that this children's book can be used to introduce the topic to young children in an age-appropriate way. This book covers topics pertinent to children such as difficulties in school and visits to the doctor. In writing this story, we did not set out to mention every medical complication that may be experienced by individuals with this condition, but rather to address those which impact young children most.

- This book is intended for children with 47, XXX (Trisomy X syndrome or Triple X) between the ages of 5 and 12 but can be read with individuals of any age.
- This is a story that a parent and child should read together.
- Talking about chromosomal variation is not a one-time event. Parents should expect to have many conversations with their child about this topic. This book can help with that discussion.
- Parents should invite their child to ask questions while reading this story. We hope that this story will encourage discussion between parent and child.
- We understand that not all girls with 47, XXX have the same experiences. For instance, not all children will require occupational therapy or have social-emotional problems. It is at the discretion of the parents to decide which details to include or omit for their child.

Enjoy!

"Eliiizaaabeth!" she hears her mom yell up the stairs. It's time to wake up for school. Sleepy, Elizabeth says to her mother, "OK, OK, I'm coming." Elizabeth sits up in bed, stretches and yawns. She has a big day ahead of her! As she stands up, she hears another voice in the hallway -- this time it's her sister. "Come on, Liz! You're going to make me late again!" Elizabeth leaves her room and heads downstairs. "Leave me alone, Megan. I'm awake," she grumbles.

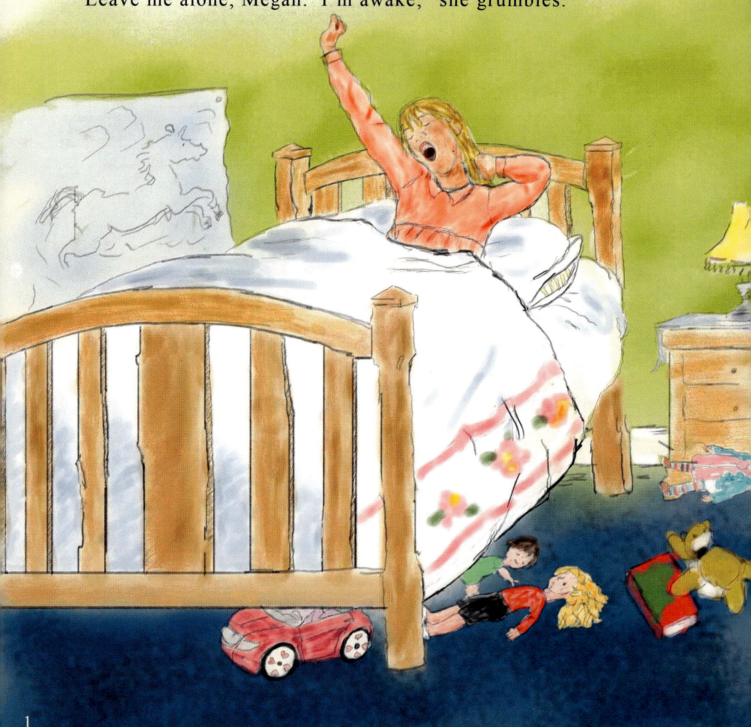

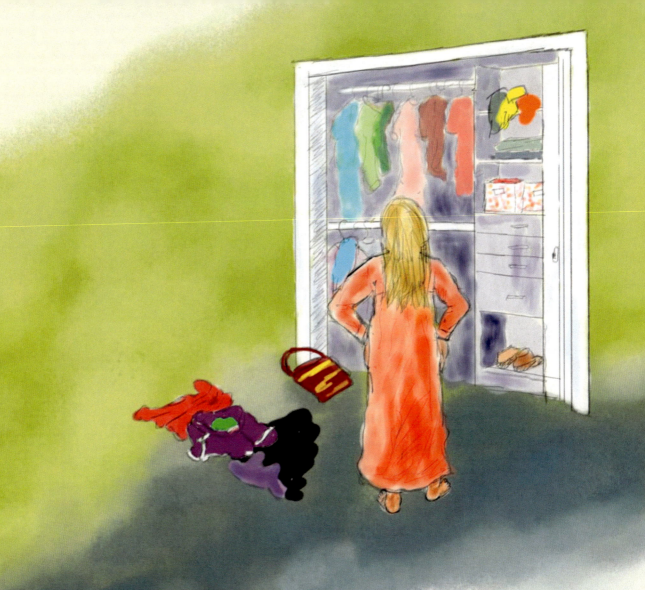

Elizabeth needs to get ready fast. She gobbles down her cereal and ignores her sister's mean looks from across the table. As she runs back upstairs, her mom yells, "Don't forget to brush your teeth!" She hates brushing her teeth.

Back in her room, it's hard to decide what to wear. Sometimes her clothes feel weird on her skin. She sees her toys and wishes she could play with them. "Liz! Come on," her sister yells. "I know! I'm coming, Meg!" she yells back. She slips on her red T-shirt, grabs her backpack and runs downstairs.

On the way to school, Elizabeth sits in the backseat while her mom and sister talk about something silly. Elizabeth stares out the window. She is still upset about how Megan yelled at her that morning. "She doesn't get it," she thinks. "Megan doesn't understand that I have to do things my own way." You see, Elizabeth is a little different. Elizabeth has an extra X. She has a condition called Trisomy X or Triple X.

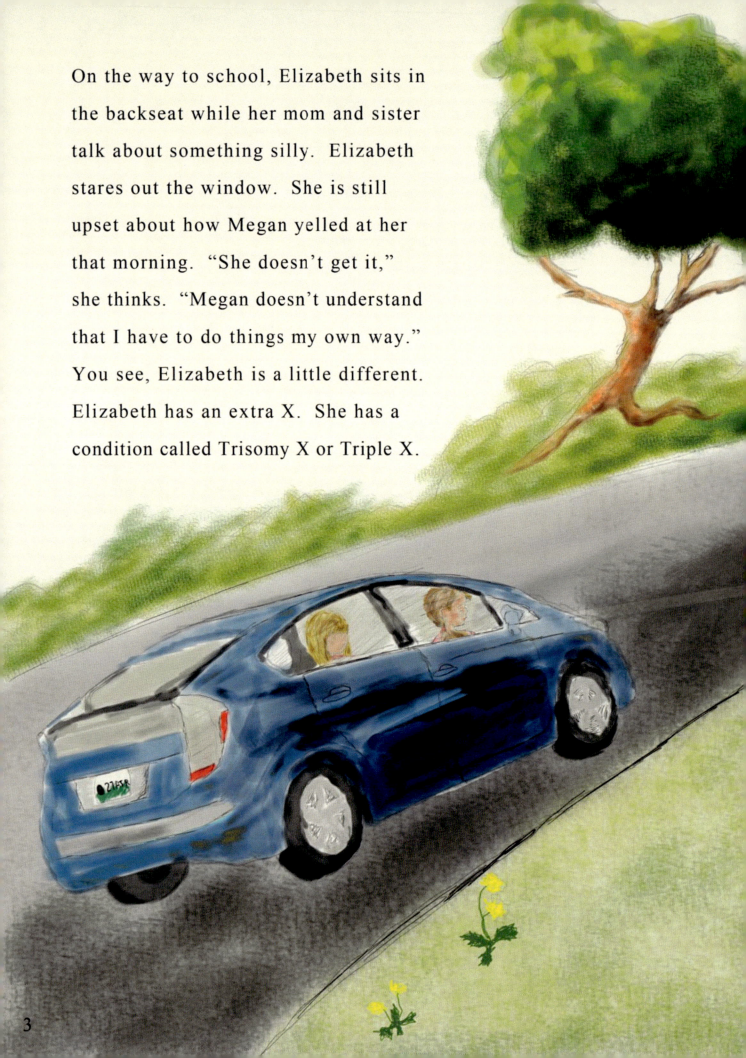

It all starts with genes. These genes are not the jeans you wear. These genes are the ones that run in families. Genes are in every cell of the body. They are the instructions that tell the body how to grow, what to look like and how to think and act. Genes are important and everyone has them, lots of them! Genes make people unique and different from one another. Without genes, people would be just faceless, brainless blobs of goo!

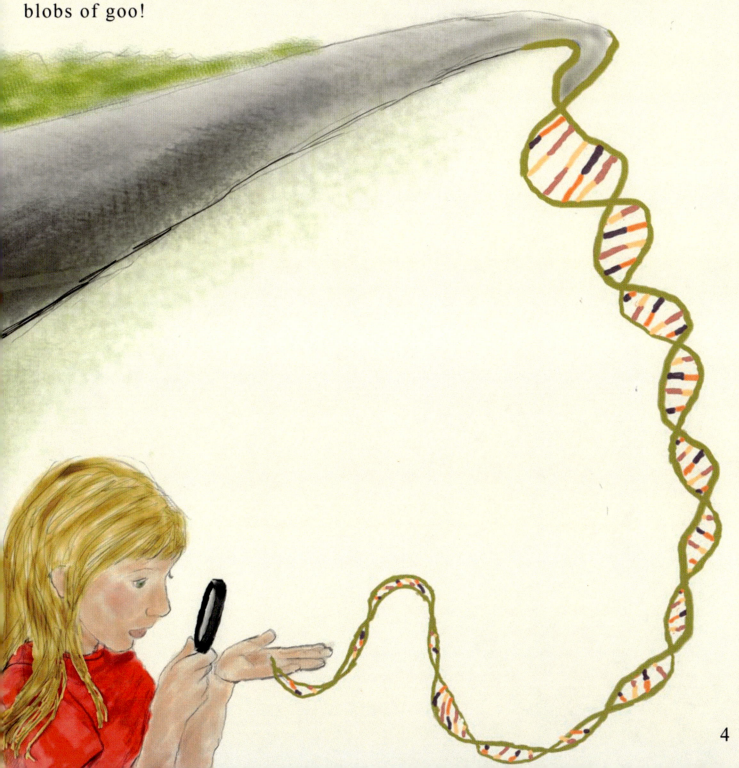

In the body, genes come in bundles called chromosomes. A chromosome holds a bundle of genes, just like a book holds a bundle of pages. There are too many genes to have just one chromosome, so people usually have 46 chromosomes to hold all of their genes. Chromosomes and genes are there from the beginning, when a baby is made. Half of the chromosomes come from your mom and the other half come from your dad. That's why kids look and act a little bit like both of their parents.

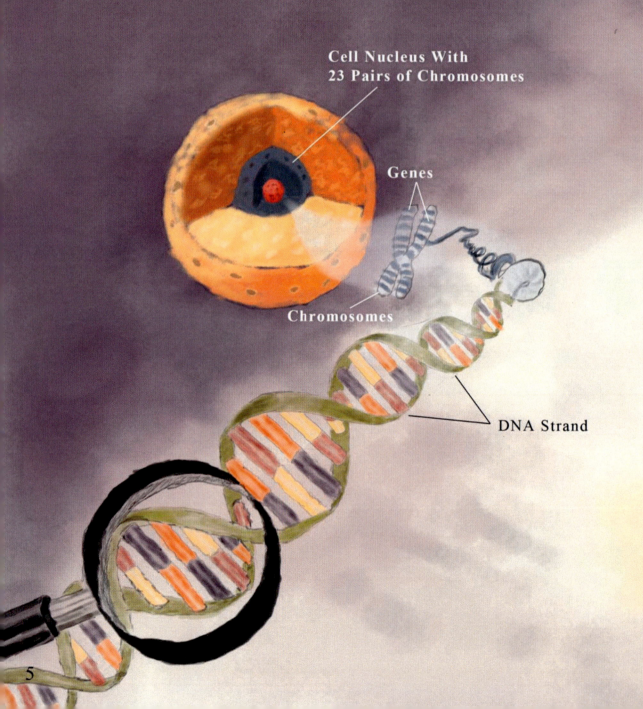

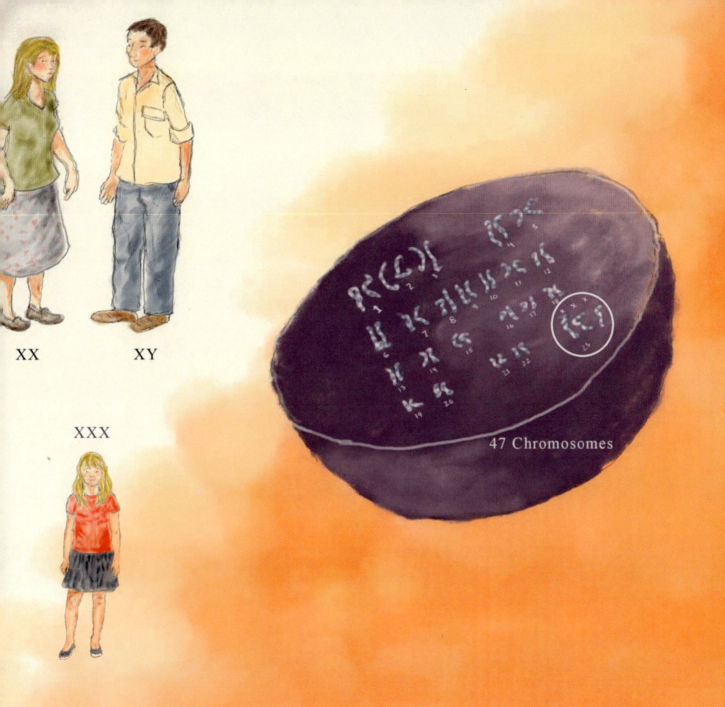

Usually, people have 46 chromosomes. Two chromosomes, the X and Y, are different from the rest. It's these X and Y chromosomes that make boys and girls different. Girls usually have two X chromosomes. Elizabeth is a girl who is a little different. She was born with an extra X chromosome, her extra X. So instead of having just two Xs like most girls, Elizabeth has three X chromosomes.

When a girl has three X chromosomes, it's called Triple X or Trisomy X. Having an extra X chromosome means Elizabeth has extra genes in her body.

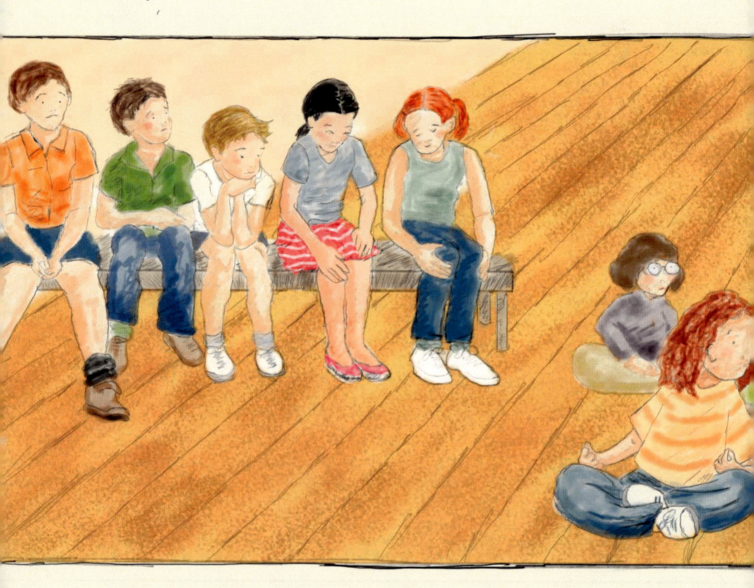

Triple X isn't a sickness like a cold that you can catch from other people. Elizabeth was just born with an extra chromosome. She isn't the only girl with Triple X either. There are other girls with extra Xs. Some of them have the same challenges as Elizabeth but some don't. Elizabeth is not ashamed of her extra X; that's just the way she is. She was made with blond hair, green eyes, rosy cheeks, and an extra X!

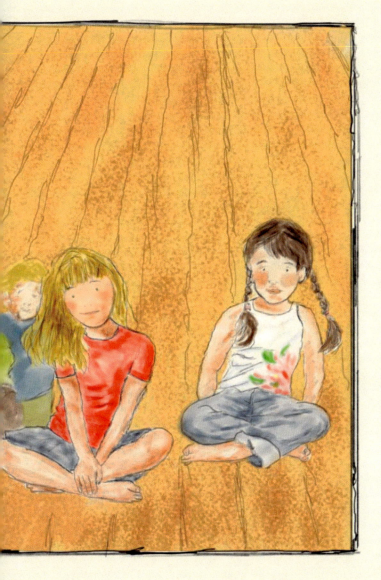

No one can tell she has an extra X chromosome just by looking at her. She looks just like the other girls. But inside her brain, sometimes her extra X chromosome makes her feel different. Sometimes having an extra X can make things harder for her, like reading or doing school work. That's what her sister doesn't understand. She doesn't get that Elizabeth is different. She has an extra X and that means she has to do things a different way sometimes.

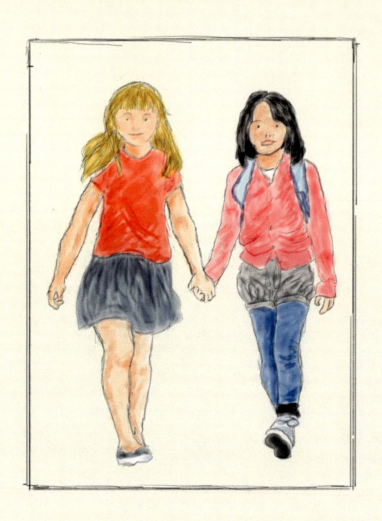

Elizabeth's mom drives up to her school. Elizabeth hops out of the car and sees other girls in her class. "Bye, Mom." She catches up with one of the girls. Elizabeth and Nancy walk to class and talk about their weekends. Nancy went to the zoo with her family and saw a big giraffe. Elizabeth wants to tell Nancy about the time she went to the zoo, but before she can put the words together, Nancy is talking about something else. Oh well. Elizabeth listens and laughs along with her friend.

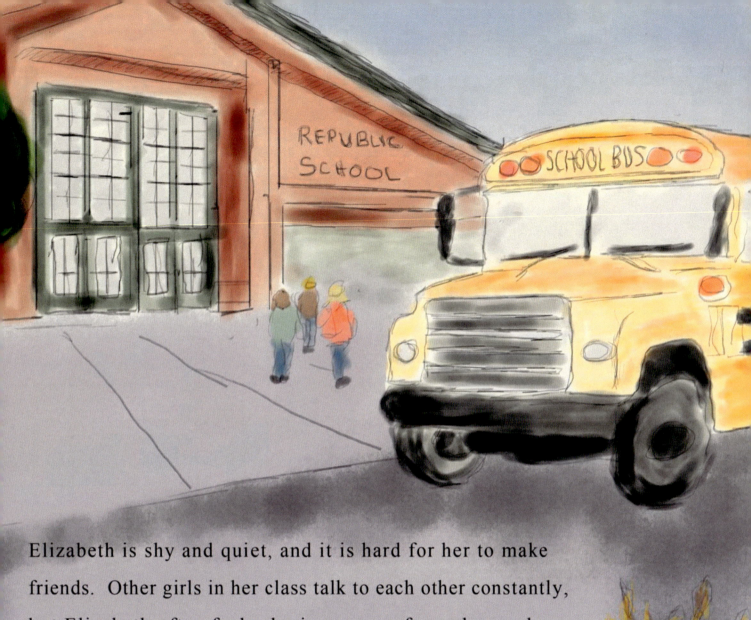

Elizabeth is shy and quiet, and it is hard for her to make friends. Other girls in her class talk to each other constantly, but Elizabeth often feels shy in groups of people, so she sits quietly. Some girls in her class don't take the time to get to know her. But the ones who do find that Elizabeth can be a really good friend! She is a nice person and is fun to be around!

The girls go into their classroom and find their seats. Elizabeth's teacher is named Ms. Adams. Elizabeth sometimes needs extra help because it's harder for her to learn and remember things. Ms. Adams gives the class 10 minutes to write a paragraph about their weekends. Elizabeth gets frustrated. She can't decide what to write about or how to start. Before she knows it, time is up and her page is blank! She is smart and can learn, just like other kids, but sometimes she has to work a little harder because of her extra X.

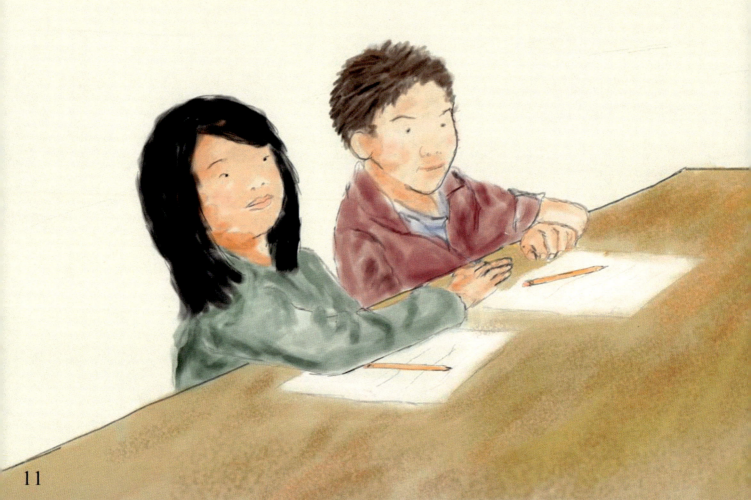

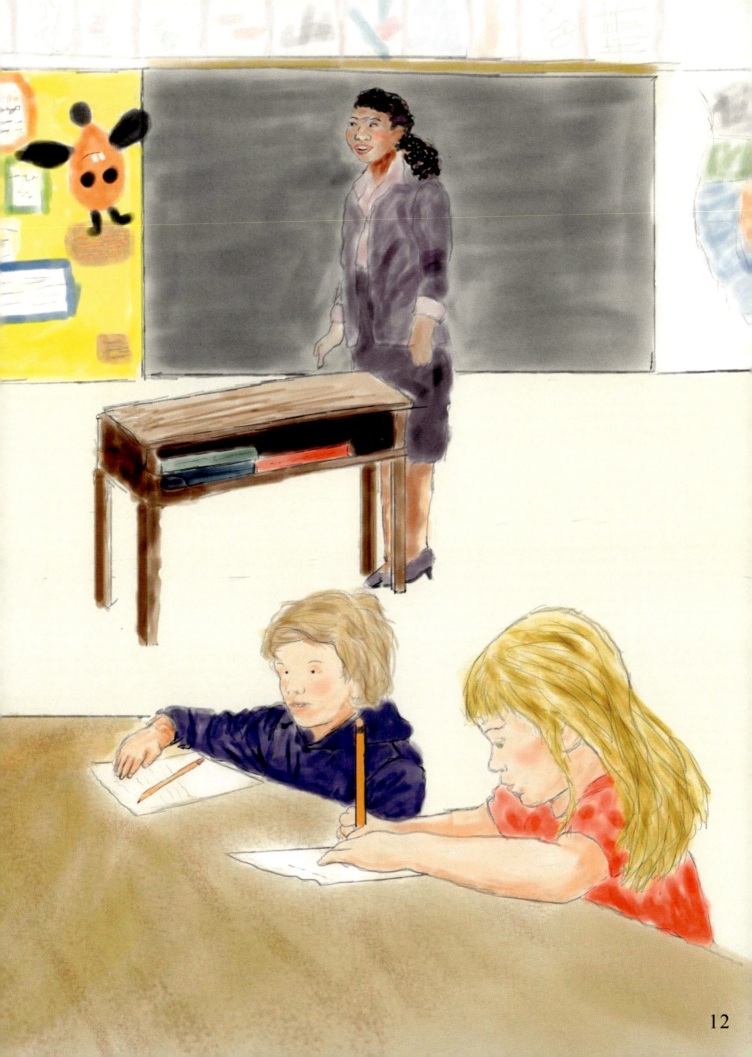

After lunch, Elizabeth leaves her class to see a speech therapist. Her speech therapist helps her learn to speak more easily. Sometimes she can't think of the word she means, or people speak too quickly for her to keep up. Other times, it's like a word gets caught in her brain, like when she wanted to talk about the zoo. In speech therapy Elizabeth practices saying these words. The more she practices, the better she gets!

Elizabeth meets with an occupational therapist at school too. Occupational therapy helps Elizabeth practice using her hands to do things that are hard for her, like handwriting and buttoning. She likes to work on her drawings. Elizabeth imagines all sorts of things to draw and is the best artist in her whole class! And the more she practices, the better she gets!

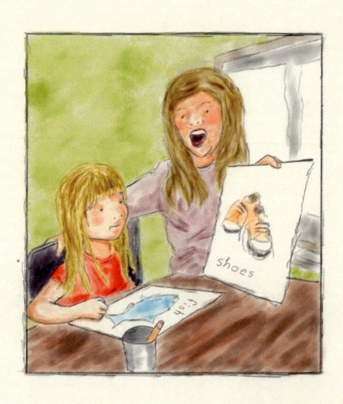 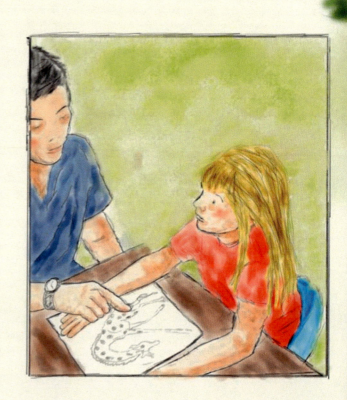

The school bell rings - recess! She likes taking a break from class and being outside. She and Nancy go to the usual spot where they play on the playground. Elizabeth looks up and sees two boys playing tag, and they are running towards her! Nervous and breathing hard, Elizabeth is glad when the boys swerve just before running into her. "Hey! Watch it!" Nancy yells. It takes a while for Elizabeth to calm down. She feels overwhelmed by the noise of everyone running around. She walks away from the others to sit by herself and calm down. She closes her eyes and catches her breath. That's better.

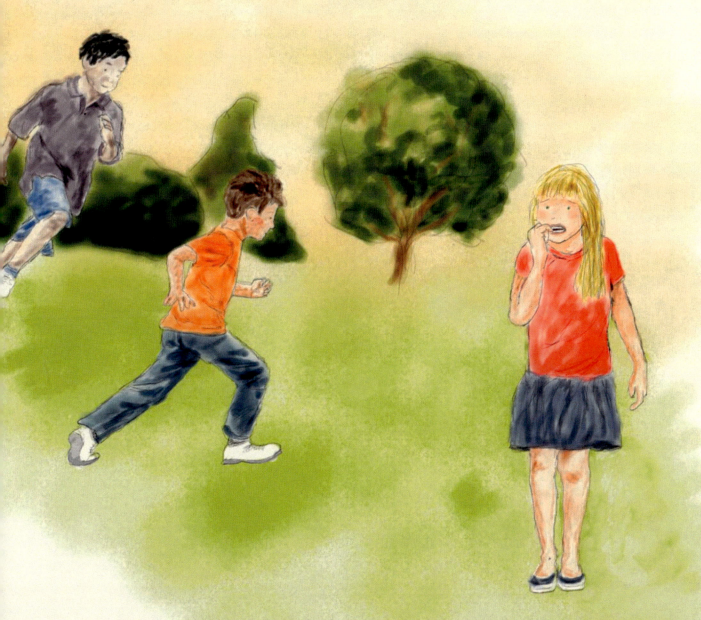

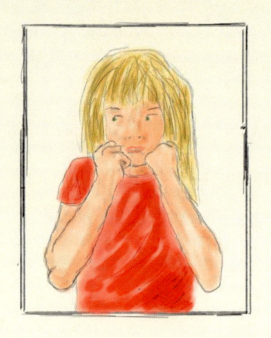
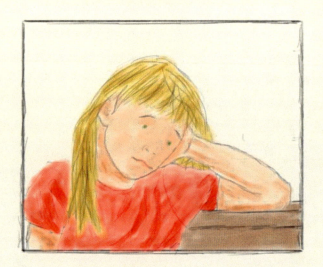
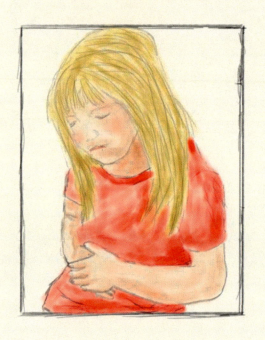

Sometimes Elizabeth feels nervous, worried or scared. She doesn't know where these feelings come from, but they sneak into her brain and make her feel like something bad is going to happen. Sometimes these feelings make her stomach hurt. When Elizabeth gets these feelings, she takes a deep breath and reminds herself that she is safe. Her counselor taught her to use tricks, like counting, to calm down. Sometimes the tricks work but sometimes they don't. The more she uses these tricks the better she is at pushing away worried thoughts. It's a different way of doing things, but it works for Elizabeth.

Ring! "Back to class," Nancy says. The second part of the day is harder for Elizabeth. Her extra X sometimes makes it hard for her to concentrate. She takes medication to help her pay attention, but it's tough at the end of the day. Elizabeth tries to listen to her teacher. It is easier to pay attention when they learn interesting things or get to use the computer. Today, the teacher is talking about something boring. She starts looking around and thinking about something else.

When school is over, the bell rings and Elizabeth snaps back to reality. "See you tomorrow, class," Ms. Adams says as the sudents get their stuff to go home.

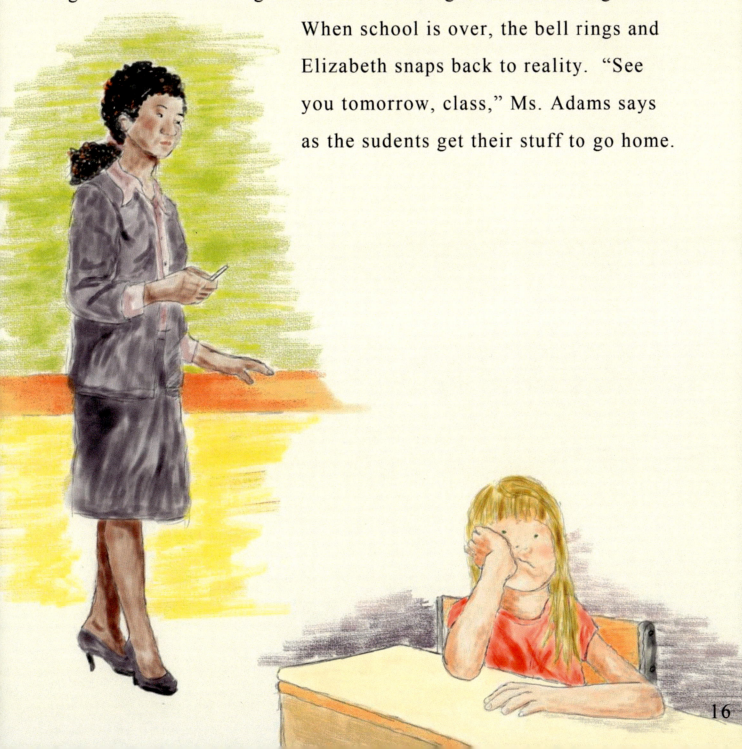

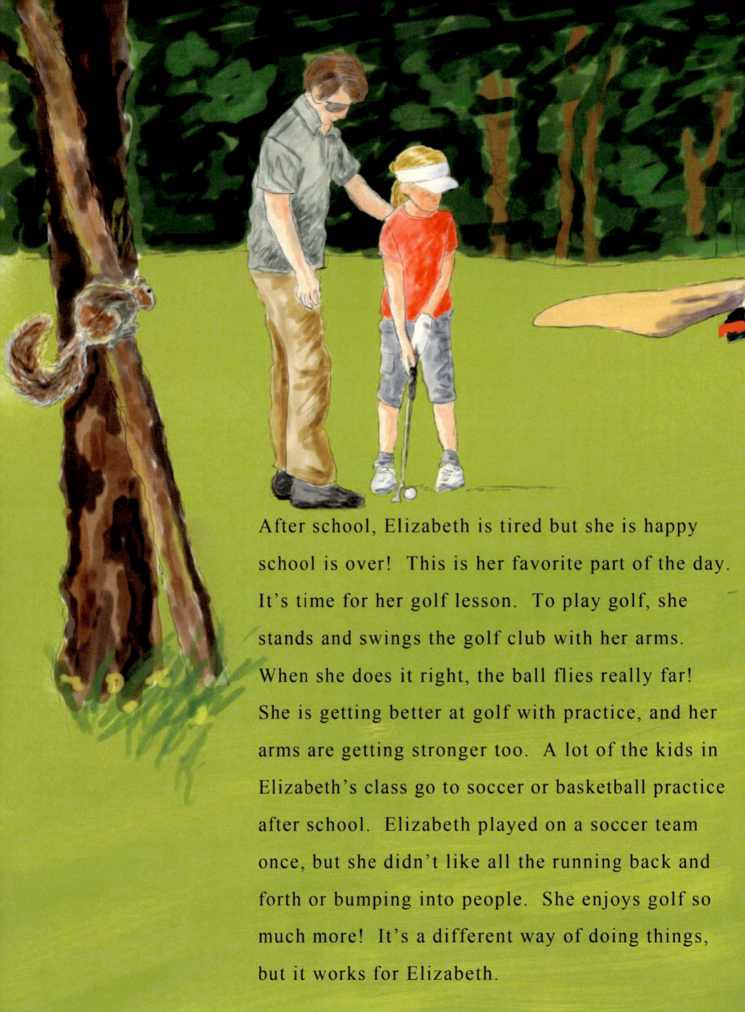

After school, Elizabeth is tired but she is happy school is over! This is her favorite part of the day. It's time for her golf lesson. To play golf, she stands and swings the golf club with her arms. When she does it right, the ball flies really far! She is getting better at golf with practice, and her arms are getting stronger too. A lot of the kids in Elizabeth's class go to soccer or basketball practice after school. Elizabeth played on a soccer team once, but she didn't like all the running back and forth or bumping into people. She enjoys golf so much more! It's a different way of doing things, but it works for Elizabeth.

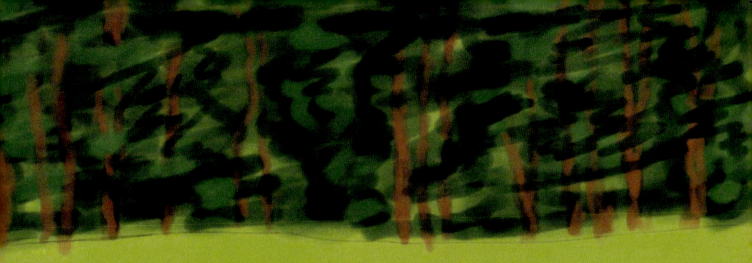

Tired from golf practice, Elizabeth walks to the parking lot. Her mom is picking her up to take her to her doctor's office. She sees her waving from her car. She smiles and waves back. "Hi, Mom," Elizabeth says. Her mom starts the car and says, "Hi, honey. How was your day?" Elizabeth says "Good." Her mom asks her questions about her day, but Elizabeth has trouble remembering the details. When she looks inside her backpack she finds the homework she forgot to turn in. "Uh-oh."

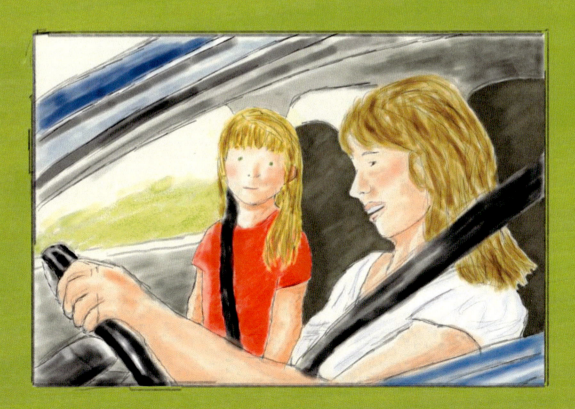

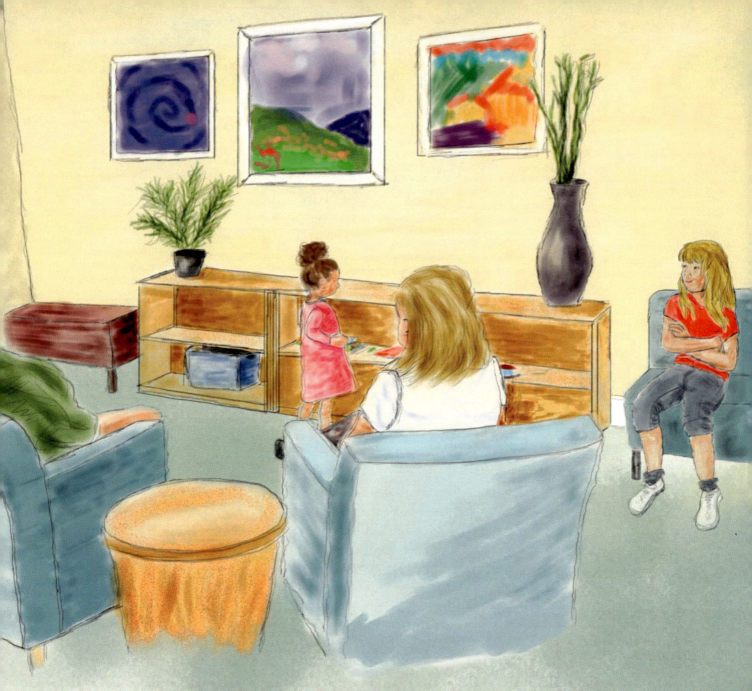

When Elizabeth and her mom get to the doctor's office, they sit in the waiting room. Elizabeth stares at the paintings on the wall. "These paintings are so ugly," she tells her mom with a laugh. "Elizabeth, don't be rude," she says, but she laughs too. Elizabeth has been in this waiting room many times before. Since Elizabeth has an extra X, she has to go to the doctor a little more than other kids. She doesn't go to the doctor because she is sick; she goes so the doctor can make sure she is healthy.

Finally, the nurse takes them back to the exam room. Elizabeth sits on the doctor's table. The doctor comes in and has Elizabeth lie down. She looks at her body, listens to her heart and looks into her ears. She pushes on her stomach which makes her laugh. "That tickles!" The doctor asks, "Elizabeth, do you know why you have to come to the doctor?" She takes a second to think. "Because I have an extra X? "That's right, Elizabeth. Girls with Triple X can be tall, sometimes have weaker muscles and need extra help in school," the doctor explains.

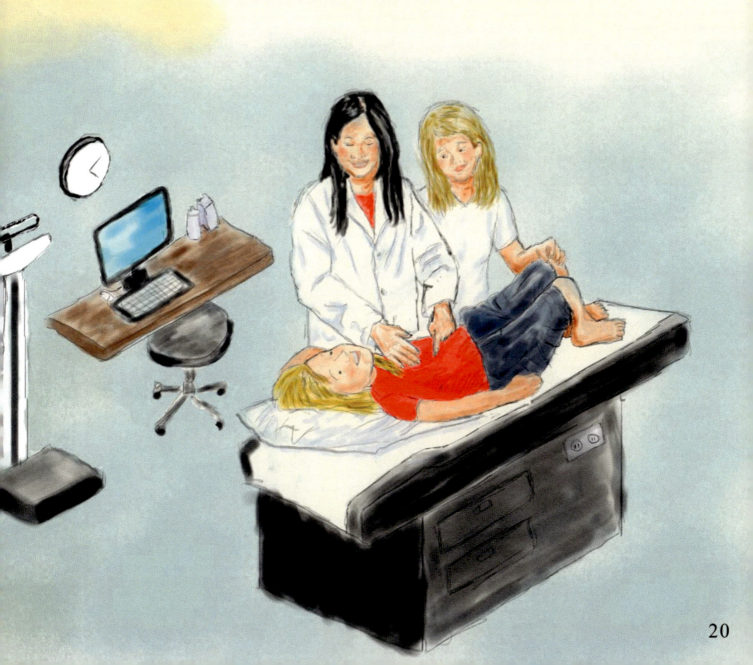

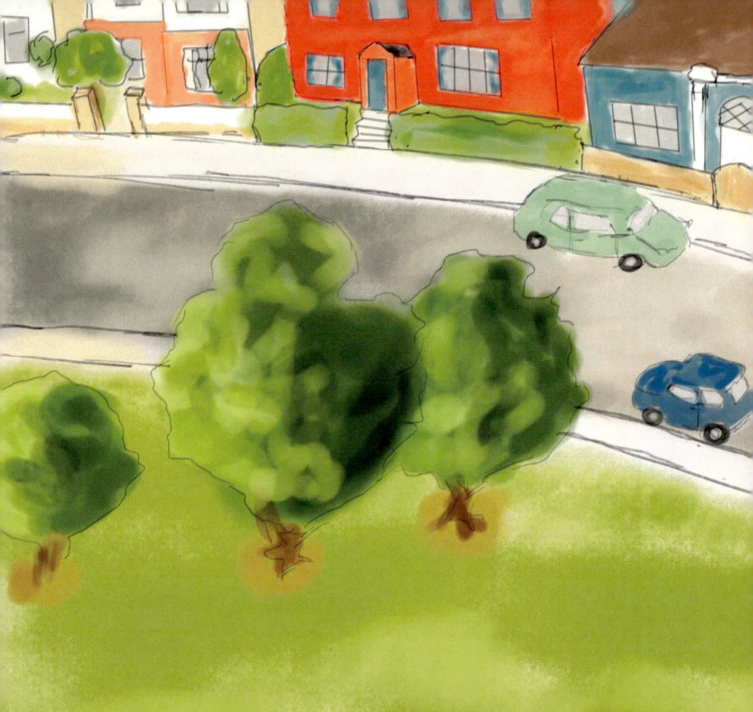

The doctor also tells Elizabeth that her extra X can make it harder for her to make decisions and plan ahead. "Having an extra X can sometimes make girls say or do things without thinking," she says. The doctor reminds Elizabeth how important it is to make safe decisions. If Elizabeth is not sure if a choice is a good one, she should ask an adult who she trusts, like her mom, dad, teacher or doctor. It's a different way of doing things, but it works for Elizabeth.

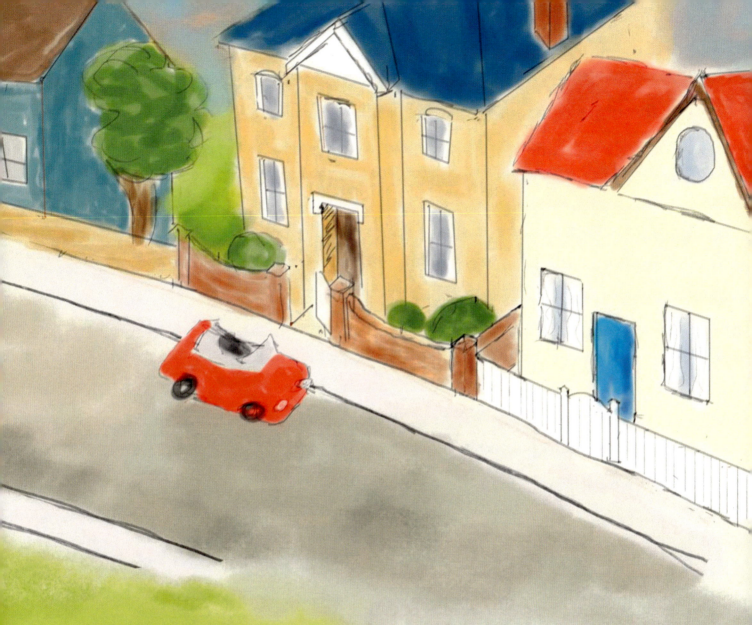

On the way home, Elizabeth stares out the car window and thinks about the future. Elizabeth is not sure what she wants to be when she grows up. There are so many things to choose from! She could be a farmer, or a teacher, or an inventor, or an artist. She could be an astronaut and live on Mars!

Someday, Elizabeth might want to be a mother and have kids. Elizabeth can be a mother when she grows up, but because of her extra X, she should talk to a doctor when she is thinking about having children. It's a different way of doing things, but it works for Elizabeth.

Back at home, Elizabeth and her family sit at the table for dinner. Megan blabs about her day. Elizabeth is too tired to listen. She wants to finish eating so she can play on the computer. Elizabeth's dad asks her about her day. She takes a second to think. "Um...Well..." "Come on, Liz, I don't have all day," her sister says with a mean grin. Elizabeth has had enough. Unable to control her feelings, she stands up from the table and yells, "Uhh! I can't stand you, Megan!" Then she runs upstairs to her bedroom and slams the door.

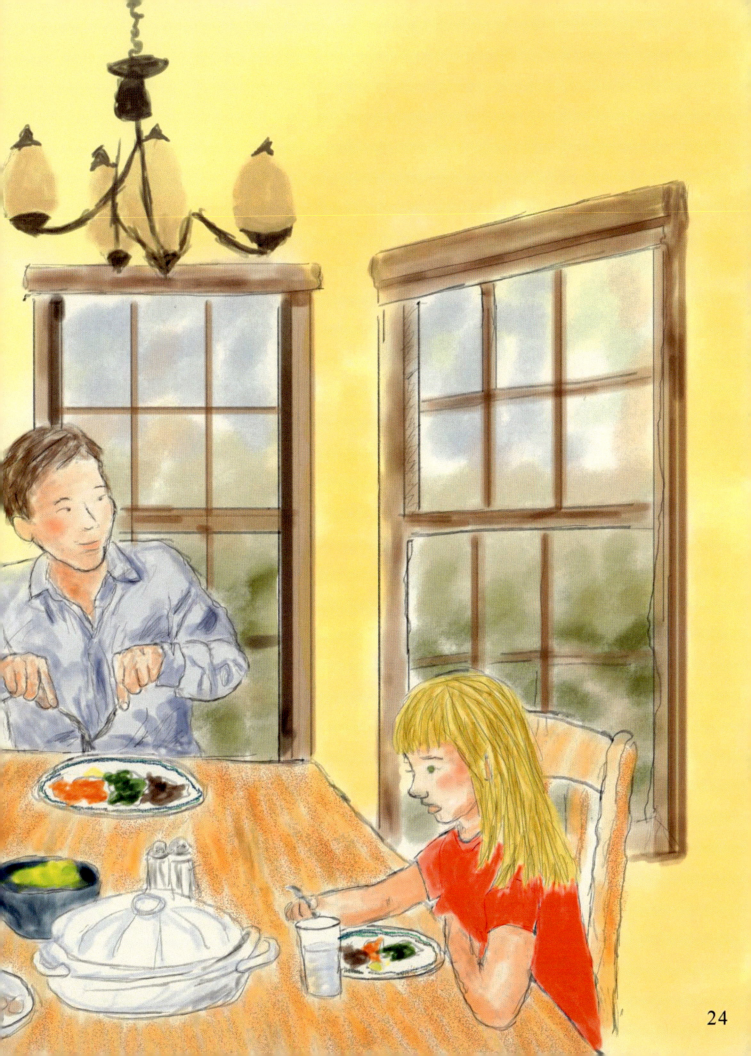

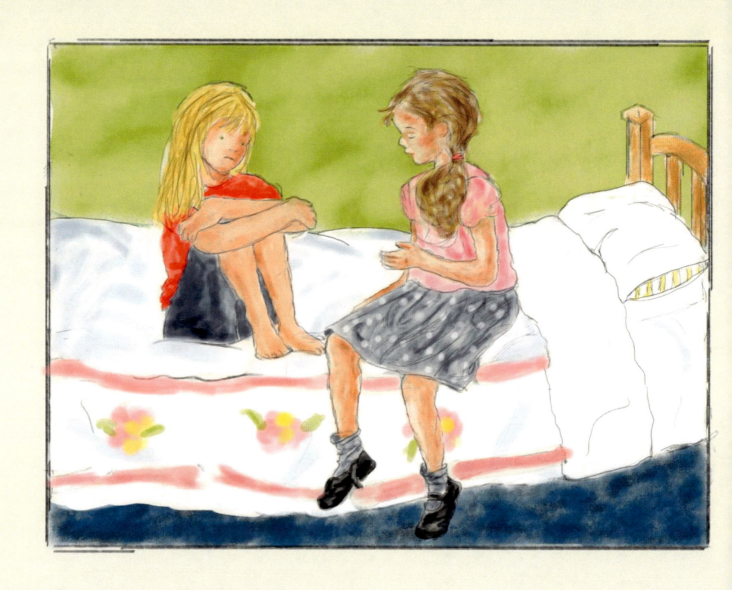

Elizabeth feels mad and frustrated. "Why does she have to be so mean to me? Doesn't she understand that things aren't as easy for me as they are for her?" Just then, the door opens. It's Megan. "I came to say sorry," she says. "I didn't mean to make you so upset. I was just teasing." "Megan, you tease me too much. I'm different from you and I have to do things my own way." "I know. I'm sorry. It's important for you to be able to do things your own way," Megan says. "I'll try to be more patient with you. I love you, little sister." Elizabeth smiles. "Yeah. I love you too, Meg."

It has been a long day. Elizabeth's mom and dad tuck her into bed. They tell her they love her and close her bedroom door. As she drifts off to sleep, she thinks about her extra X. Triple X is really just a small part of who Elizabeth is. Her extra X makes her unique and different, just like all of her talents and traits make her unique and different. Her extra X is just one of many, many things that make Elizabeth who she is. When she was made, she ended up with an extra X. It's a different way of doing things, but it works for Elizabeth.

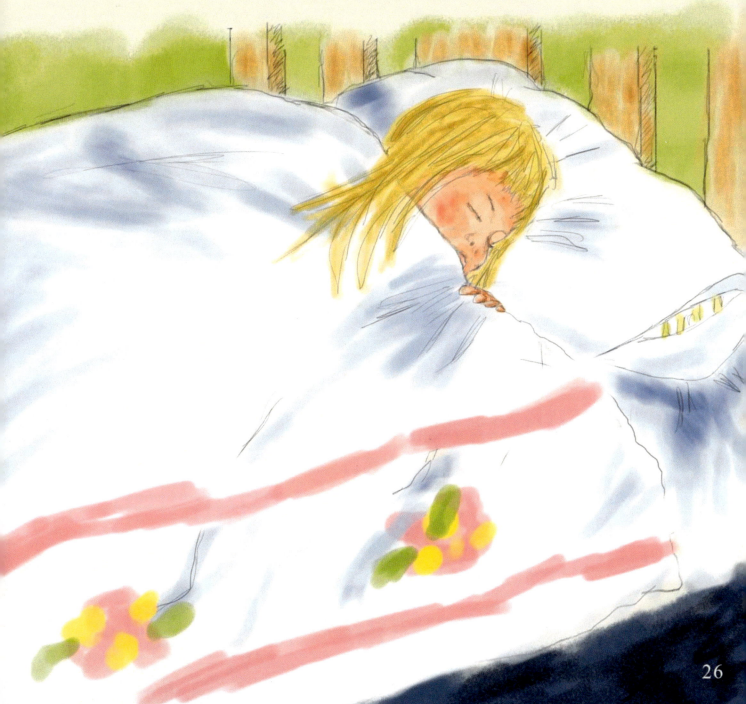

The end.

Acknowledgements

Creating this series of books would not have been possible without the time and dedication of many people who had a hand in bringing it to life.

Firstly, I am indebted to the many parents of children with X and Y chromosome variations who took the time to read the books between the time of their inception through to their final stages. The feedback they provided was so important in helping to craft the stories into ones that so many children will be able to relate to as they flip through these pages. Thank you for your time, wisdom and enthusiam.

I would also like to thank Susan Howell, Dr. Nicole Tartaglia and their colleagues at the eXtraordinarY kids Clinic, whose expertise and advice guided me through the creation of these books. Thank you for your patience, your encouragement and for reading these books almost as many times as I have.

Many thanks go to Suzanne Hayes, the illustrator of this series of books. With her creativity and talents, she was able to take my words and bring them to life in full color images. Her efforts turned my stories into children's books. I appreciate every minute of hard work she devoted to making this project a success.

My editor, Alexa McGuinness, deserves a great deal of thanks for remembering the grammar rules that I didn't and taking the time to read through every line of my books looking for them.

Finally, I would like to thank my family for supporting me in everything that I do and lending names to so many of my characters.

Arlie Colvin
Author

About the author

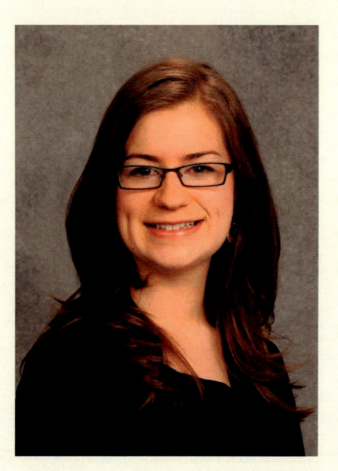

Born and raised in Muskegon, MI, Arlie Colvin received her Bachelor of Science from the University of Michigan. She attended the University of Colorado Denver to pursue her Master of Science in genetic counseling. She became interested in writing children's books for kids with X and Y chromosome variations while working for the eXtraordinarY Kids Clinic at Children's Hospital Colorado as a graduate student. Arlie enjoys spending time with her family, hiking and painting. She hopes to have a long career as a genetic counselor and children's book author, and impact many people along the way.

About the illustrator

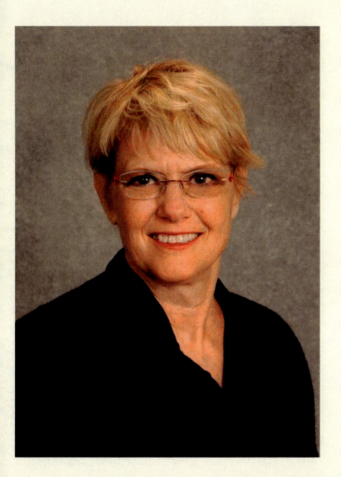

After a long career as an outdoor clothing designer and patternmaker, Suzanne Hayes returned to school at the University of Colorado Denver. She became interested in pursuing a Masters Degree in Medical Illustration in order to combine her artistic side with her love of the sciences. When she is not exploring the outdoors, she works hard at her art. She has especially enjoyed learning digital painting and drawing, using the storyline to come up with scenes that are illustative, corlorful and fun. Suzanne looks forward to having a long and successful career exploring the medical and biological sciences through illustration.

Made in the USA
Monee, IL
03 December 2020